Super Foods Originality

Joseph Anderson

Table of content

Introduction

We all in all find out about the various wonderful food assortments that are perfect to eat and bravo. We by and large learn about eating natural items, vegetables, and nuts.

However, that is a significant once-over to sort out, and wouldn't it be able to be more direct to have two or three super food assortments that you can consistently go to? To help you in your endeavors to lead a strong lifestyle and a sound life you can use the overview assembled as an expedient reference once-over of 9 superfood sources.

Apples

Apples are an incredible nourishment for some reasons including the capacity to diminish the gamble or coronary illness, certain tumors, hypertension, and type-2 diabetes. They likewise benefit the respiratory framework by forestalling cellular breakdown in the lungs and asthma.

By consuming apples your body gets fiber, potassium, and cancer prevention agents, like Vitamin C and polyphenols. Concentrates on a show that the genuine advantage comes from the synergistic association between these fixings.

To exploit apples for your wellbeing, eat a wide assortment and ensure that you eat the strip, which contains a few times a greater number of cell reinforcements than within. As is commonly said, eat an apple daily.

Avocados

At the point when you need to assist your body with engrossing additional supplements from the food varieties you eat, have an avocado as well. Fat solvent phytonutrients, similar to beta-carotene, are all the more handily consumed by the body due to the monounsaturated fat in the avocado.

Avocados additionally assist you with holding your weight down since they assist you with feeling full, which sets off your body to quit eating. They are calorie rich at 48 calories for each ounce, so for best outcomes eat 33% to a one-a portion of an avocado a few times each week.

Dull Chocolate

At the point when you need a little guilty pleasure with your well-being food, attempt dim chocolate. It contains loads of polyphenols which lower circulatory strain and is a characteristic calming. You ought to remember that circulatory strain bringing down characteristics are just in dim chocolate, but not in its cousin, milk chocolate.

In 2000 a review distributed by the American Journal of Clinical Nutrition showed that the impact on the bloodstream from high flavanol cocoa was like taking low-portion headache medicine. This implies that dim chocolate might be utilized to deal with sicknesses like minor agonies or migraines.

For the best outcomes utilize Newman's Own Sweet Dart Chocolate, as Dr. Pratt has found it has more polyphenols than some other dull chocolate he has found. Like avocado, chocolate is high in calories, so go for at least 100 calories every day.

Olive Oil

There has been a lot of conversation recently about the advantages of the Mediterranean eating routine. Well, olive oil is one of the fundamental parts of that eating regimen and its advantages are remarkable. It is an extraordinary substitute for different oils and fats and has been displayed to lessen the gamble of bosom and colon malignant growth, lower circulatory strain, and work on the wellbeing of your cardiovascular framework.

For best outcomes take a tablespoon daily of additional virgin olive oil that is cold squeezed and greenish in variety. This green variety assists you with spotting elevated degrees of polyphenols.

Garlic

One more part of the Mediterranean eating routine, Garlic is perfect for your cardiovascular framework. By eating garlic consistently, you can diminish your circulatory strain, fatty substance levels, and your LDL(bad) cholesterol. Garlic likewise has mitigating specialists and anti-toxin properties.

To snatch all the medical advantages of garlic, eat one clove a few times each week. Crude garlic is ideal, however, cooked is great as well. Remember that dried garlic and garlic supplements don't have similar advantages as new garlic.

Honey

Honey isn't much of the time seen in many arrangements of good food sources, however, don't let that fool you. Eating honey every day expands the measures of cell reinforcement in the blood, assists with forestalling clogging, and decreases cholesterol and pulse.

Assuming you are running almost out of energy, go after the honey, not sugar. Honey improves at keeping up with glucose and energy than different sugars. Furthermore, pick dim honey over light ones, since they are higher in cancer prevention agents and flavor. One to two teaspoons a few times each week ought to get the job done.

Kiwis

If you need outrageous amounts of Vitamin C and E that can decrease the hazard of asthma, osteoarthritis, and colon malignant growth, and lift your resistant framework, then, at that point, get a kiwi or two. A fascinating point to remember is that dietary vitamin E seems to bring down the gamble of Alzheimer's, and by devouring kiwis, you get vitamin E without the calories that most other vitamin e rich food sources contain, similar to nuts and oils.

Another heavenly fixing is lutein, which brings down the gamble waterfalls and macular degeneration. To get every one of the above benefits and diminish the gamble of blood clumps, then consume one kiwi, a few times each week.

Onions

For the advantages of onions, you can simply rehash the advantages of garlic, since they are something similar.

Attempt to eat dishes containing onions something like three times each week, and ensure that you let the onion sit for 5 to 10 minutes after you cut it open. Assuming you apply heat too early you will deactivate the thiopropanal sulfoxide, which is the substance in the onion that gives us the most heart benefits. Furthermore, recall the sharper the onion, the better it is for you.

Pomegranates

Pomegranates are loaded with lots of phytochemicals like potassium, which is perfect for bringing down your circulatory strain. Concentrates additionally recommend that pomegranates can slow the movement of prostate disease and decrease the gamble of atherosclerosis.

Rather than battling with the little thick seeds to get your portion of pomegranate, attempt four to eight ounces of 100 percent squeeze a few times each week. Make certain to avoid juices with added sugar.

Section 1

Nutrition - The Super Foods That Keep You Healthy

Prepare to encounter a volume of data on the best food sources on the planet.

Here is a rundown of the main ten super food sources that most wellbeing specialists settle on. You ought to tell everybody you are familiar with these food varieties and appreciate them at your next feast. From leafy foods to entire grains, nuts, beans, and vegetables, this power-stuffed wholesome stock will bring you into the greatest long periods of your life and then some.

Organic products

Melon

Just a fourth of melon gives practically all the vitamin A required in one day. Since the beta-carotene in a melon converts to vitamin A, you get the two supplements on the double. These vision-reinforcing supplements might assist with lessening the gamble of creating waterfalls.

Like an orange, melon is additionally a superb wellspring of L-ascorbic acid, which helps our invulnerable framework. It is likewise being a decent wellspring of vitamin B6, dietary fiber, folate, niacin, and potassium, which keeps up with great glucose levels and digestion. This light orange power natural product might assist with decreasing our gamble of coronary illness, stroke, and disease.

Blueberries

These somewhat sweet (and once in a while tart) berries offer a high ability to obliterate free extremists that can cause malignant growth. Low in calories, they offer cell reinforcement phytonutrients called anthocyanidins, which upgrade the impacts of L-ascorbic acid. These cell reinforcements might assist with forestalling waterfalls, glaucoma, varicose veins, hemorrhoids, peptic ulcers, coronary illness, and malignant growth.

Vegetables

3: Tomatoes

Tomatoes assist us with battling coronary illness and tumors like colorectal, prostate, bosom, endometrial, lung, and disease of the pancreas. Tomatoes are likewise great wellsprings of L-ascorbic acid, A, and K. In a recent report, it was found that tomato squeeze alone can assist with lessening blood coagulating.

New, natural tomatoes convey threefold the amount of the disease battling carotenoid lycopene. Indeed, even natural ketchup is preferable for you over customary ketchup! Search for tomato glue and sauces that contain the entire tomato (counting strips) since you will ingest 75% more lycopene and very nearly twice how much beta-carotene.

4: Sweet Potatoes

As a brilliant wellspring of nutrients, A, C, and manganese, yams are likewise a decent wellspring of copper, dietary fiber, vitamin B6, potassium, and iron. The people who are smokers or inclined to recycle smoke might benefit incredibly from this root vegetable that safeguards us against emphysema.

For an exceptional treat, 3D shape a cooked yam and cut a banana. Then daintily pour maple syrup over the top and add a scramble or two of cinnamon. Add slashed pecans for a considerably better kick.

5: Spinach and Kale

A disease contender and cardio-partner, spinach and kale top the rundown, all things considered. Similar to broccoli, they give a brilliant wellspring of vitamin An and C. Kale is a shockingly decent wellspring of calcium at 25% per cup, bubbled. Vitamin K is plentifully tracked down in spinach also, with practically 200% of the Daily Value accessible, to assist with lessening bone misfortune.

Entire Grains

6: Whole Grain Bread, Pasta, and Brown Rice

Whether it's bread or pasta, the principal thing to check for while buying
entire grain bread and pasta are to ensure it is 100 percent entire grain.

Make sure to take a look at the rundown of fixings on the bundle. For instance, search for the specific expression "entire wheat flour" as one of the principal fixings recorded in entire wheat bread. If it's not recorded thusly, then it's not the entire grain.
Wheat grain is a malignant growth battling grain that likewise assists us with controlling our defecations.

Earthy colored rice is likewise a preferable decision over the refined grain (white rice) for a similar explanation as picking entire wheat bread. Entire wheat flour or earthy colored rice that transforms into white flour or white rice annihilates between 50-90% of vitamin B3, vitamin B1, vitamin B6, manganese, phosphorus, iron, and the entirety of the dietary fiber and fundamental unsaturated fats we want.

In any event, when handled white flour or white rice is "improved," it isn't in a similar structure as the first natural kind. Truth be told, 11 supplements are lost and are not supplanted during the "enhancement" process!

Nuts

7: Walnuts

These nuts are loaded with omega-3 fats, which is one of the "upside" fats. A quarter cup of pecans would deal with around 90% of the omega-3s required in one day. Pecans give numerous medical advantages including cardiovascular security, better mental capability, calming benefits connecting with asthma, rheumatoid joint pain, and provocative skin illnesses like dermatitis and psoriasis. They might help against malignant growth and support the resistant framework.

Beans and Legumes

8: Black Beans and Lentils

While dark beans are a decent wellspring of fiber that can bring down cholesterol, lentils are as well. The high fiber content in both dark beans and lentils assists with keeping up with glucose levels. Likewise, a sans fat, a great protein with extra minerals and B-nutrients, dark beans and lentils top you off and don't grow your waistline.

A total, one-stop wellspring of utilizing various beans and lentils comes simply when you can find a sack of 15-bean blend (incorporates dark beans, lentils, naval force, pinto, red, kidney, and so on) at the supermarket. Consider making a flavorful soup with the expansion of tomatoes, onions, garlic, and your number one flavors with this bean blend.

Dairy

9: Skim Milk and Yogurt

Skim milk (or low-fat) assists with serious areas of strength for advancing, offering a great wellspring of calcium, vitamin D, and vitamin K. These supplements assist with safeguarding colon cells from disease-causing synthetics, and bone misfortune, headache migraines, premenstrual side effects, and youth heftiness. Ongoing investigations additionally show that overweight grown-ups get more fit, particularly around the midriff, while polishing off low-fat dairies like skim milk and yogurt.

Yogurt additionally incorporates fundamental supplements, for example, phosphorous and vitamin B2, vitamin B12, vitamin B5, zinc, potassium, and protein. Yogurt's live bacterial societies likewise give an abundance of medical advantages that might end up being useful to us live longer and fortify our invulnerable framework.

Fish

10: Salmon

Salmon is high in protein, low in absorbed fat, and high in omega-3 fats (the major unsaturated fats that are also found in those walnuts referred to previously). Salmon is a heart-decent food and is endorsed to eat something like twice consistently.

While picking salmon, it's ideal to stay away from farm raised and select wild taking everything into account. Research focuses on a show that developed salmon could cause threatening development since it could convey raised levels of malignant growth causing engineered compounds known as polychlorinated biphenyls (PCBs).

Others

Green Tea and "Power" Water

Yet not food per se, the clinical benefits of these beverages merit referring to.

Green tea has accommodating phytonutrients and lower levels of caffeine than any leftover teas. The more assessment focusing on green tea, the more clinical benefits are found. A dangerous development competitor as well, green tea has cell support influences that lower risks of bacterial or viral pollution to cardiovascular contamination, infection, stroke, periodontal disorder, and osteoporosis.

Water stacked with supplements or possibly typically further developed regular items are moreover the latest example. Some suggest a whole day's reserve of L-ascorbic corrosive while others ensure no fake sugars with a full, fruity taste.

As might be self-evident, the really ten super food assortments merit each snack (or taste). Since it is currently so clear which food assortments can help with saving your life, what's a higher need than placing assets into your prosperity?

Section 2

You Are What You Eat

Continuous dietary assessment has uncovered 14 different enhancement thick food assortments that on various events advance perfect in everyday prosperity.

Initiated "superfoods," will for the most part have fewer calories, more huge degrees of supplements and minerals, and various infection-fighting disease counteraction specialists.

Beans (vegetables), berries (especially blueberries), broccoli, green tea, nuts (especially walnuts), oranges, pumpkin, salmon, soy, spinach, tomatoes, turkey, whole grains and oats, and yogurt can all help stop and, shockingly, rearrange infections like hypertension, diabetes, Alzheimer's, and a couple of sorts of threatening development.

Besides, where one could influence a particular piece of the body, it can similarly impact the strength of other body capacities and execution, since the whole body is related.

With these 14 food sources as the underpinning of a fair, solid eating schedule, weight decrease stunts and other impermanent tasks can transform into a remnant of bygone ages in your day-to-day existence.

Then again, the shrewd effects of a lopsided eating routine are a couple and moved. Low energy levels, demeanor swings, tired continually, weight change, and an off-kilter body are two or three signs that your eating routine is inconsistent. A lopsided eating routine can make issues with the upkeep of body tissues, advancement and improvement, frontal cortex and tactile framework capacity, as well as issues with bone and muscle systems.

Results of craving integrate nonattendance of energy, bad temper, an incapacitated insusceptible structure provoking unremitting colds or responsive qualities, and mineral utilization that can set off a combination of prosperity concerns including whiteness.

In addition, since the body is related, understanding that a bothersome body will achieve an appalling soul simply gives off an impression of being genuine. Right when we support our body with these superfoods and supplement them with other enhancement thick and sound new food sources, our spirit will be vitalized and strong as a quick result.

Various state-of-the-art eats fewer carbs considering prepackaged solace food sources are horrendously ailing in various supplements and minerals, which can impact our mental restricts as well, and causes crabbiness, disturbance, and the vibe of 'being in a murkiness' continually.

Superfoods can be the reason for a sound, strong, nutritious response for reestablishing an impressive parcel of these infections and that is just a hint of something larger.

Section 3

Color Your Way to Daily Health

We should eat a great deal of different verdant food varieties reliably.

Thins down well off in results of the dirt could reduce the bet of harmful development and other continuous ailments. Verdant food sources give major supplements and minerals, fiber, and various substances that are critical for good prosperity. Most verdant food sources are ordinarily low in fat and calories and are filling.

You've probably found out about the 5 A Day for Better Health program. It gives basic strategies for adding more results of the dirt into your everyday eating plans. We truly should eat a wide variety of splendid orange/yellow, red, green, white, and blue/purple vegetables and normal items reliably.

By eating vegetables and regular item from every assortment bundle, you will benefit from the principal supplements, minerals, and fiber that every assortment pack offers that might be of some value alone and in the blend.

There are a couple of various yet clear approaches to starting coordinating vegetables and natural items into your unmistakable and most adored feasts. You can begin your day with 100 percent regular item or vegetable juice, cut bananas or strawberries on top of your cereal, or have a plate of leafy greens with lunch and an apple for a late morning snack.

Consolidate a vegetable with dinner and you at this point have around 5 cups of verdant food sources. You could make a pass by adding a piece of a normal item for a chomp or an extra vegetable at dinner.

Make it a highlight to have a go at a truly new thing to fabricate your vegetable and natural item utilization. There are innumerable choices when picking the results of the dirt. Kiwifruit, asparagus, and mango could transform into your new number one. Keep things new and charming by joining food sources developed starting from the earliest stage with different flavors and assortments, like red grapes with pineapple knots, or cucumbers and red peppers.

Begin keeping results of the dirt obvious and accessible

- you will frequently eat them more. Store cut and cleaned produce at eye-level in the ice chest, or keep a significant splendid bowl of the normal item on the table.

Section 4

Superfoods For Age-Defying Beauty

This article examines the World's Top 6 superfoods for outrageous age-contradicting brilliance.

6 superfoods for age-testing heavenliness:

Goji Berries

Goji berries, Hollywood's most boiling new food, are maybe of the most invigoratingly thick food on earth and house a staggering centralization of supplements, minerals, amino acids, phytochemicals, and basic unsaturated fats. With such an extraordinary constitution it isn't stunning they are supposed foe of developing miracles.

Beginning in Tibet and essentially liked in ordinary prescription these dried berries enjoy many noted health advantages including supporting obstruction, cutting down cholesterol, further developing vision, engaging illness cells, facilitating unhappiness, and aiding weight decrease.

Goji berries contain on numerous occasions more L-ascorbic corrosive than oranges by weight and more beta-carotene than carrots making them a brilliant wellspring of vitamin A. Alongside vitamin E and major unsaturated fats, these berries are perfect for any foe of developing and brilliance framework.

They furthermore contain polysaccharides, one of which has been found to vitalize the release of the reestablishing human advancement substance by the pituitary organ, as well as B supplements, 21 minerals, and 18 amino acids.

The most undeniable occasion of life expectancy is that of Li Qing Yuen, who lived to the age of 252. Brought into the world in 1678, he is said to have hitched on various occasions with 11 periods of any sort of future family before his end in 1930. Li Qing Yuen consumed goji berries every day.

A survey referred to in Dr. Mindell's book 'Goji: The Himalayan Health Secret', seen that 67% of elderly people that were given an ordinary piece of

the berries for quite a while experienced profound safe structure redesign and a basic improvement in soul and cheerfulness.

Aloe Vera

Dismiss Botox, Aloe Vera increases collagen creation 100% regularly for an enthusiastic, sans wrinkle synthesis and bold, exquisite skin. A conclusive Botox elective!

The inner gel of the Aloe vera leaf contains around 200 unique combinations with more than 75 enhancements. These integrate 20 minerals, 18 amino acids, and 12 supplements (even vitamin B12 - an extremely uncommon illustration of plant wellsprings of this supplement).

Aloe Vera similarly has unfriendly microbial properties combating living beings and microorganisms and houses quieting plant steroids and synthetics. Aloe Vera is known to help handling and end, support the safe system, and be significantly convincing at recovering, soaking, and re-establishing the skin, ordinarily vivifying the making of collagen.

Aloe Vera is most ideal eaten new when (you can organize immense Aloe Vera leaves which last a portion of a month refrigerated). Fix inside the gel, avoiding an outside point of view of the leaf which is a solid area for a, and blend in with natural item for a conclusive upgrading smoothie. Aloe Vera tastes truly delicate anyway a slight extreme edge, in this manner is best gotten together with the regular item.

Avocados

Avocados are smoothing and mellowing for the skin and effectively assimilated; contrasted and almond, corn, olive, and soybean oils, avocado oil has the most noteworthy skin entrance rate.

Avocado additionally contains vitamin E (superb for the skin), cancer prevention agent carotenoids, and the expert cell reinforcement glutathione that is astoundingly strong and hostile to cancer-causing potential. Elevated degrees of glutathione is found in the liver where the disposal of poisonous materials happens.

Glutathione is successful against contaminations, for example, tobacco smoke and exhaust vapor as well as bright radiation. Research is as of now investigating the expected advantages of glutathione for various circumstances

counting malignant growth, coronary illness, cognitive decline, joint pain, Parkinson's infection, dermatitis, liver problems, weighty metal harming, and AIDS.

Chlorella

The nucleic acids RNA and DNA in Chlorella (one of the greatest known wellsprings of such) direct cell development and fix and empower our bodies to use supplements all the more real, take out poisons and keep away from illness.

The development of nucleic acids in the body declines dynamically as we age, which is no question why their admission is suggested by Dr. Benjamin Frank in 'The No-Aging Diet'.

Paul Pitchford in 'Recuperating with Whole Foods' composes that 'deficient nucleic corrosive causes untimely maturing as well as debilitated resistance', Research at the Medical College of Kanazawa in Japan observed that mice that were taken care of chlorella had a 30 percent increment in life range. Renewing RNA and DNA can be vital to generally speaking wellbeing, insusceptibility, and life span.

Notwithstanding nucleic acids, chlorella is jam-loaded with nutrients, minerals, cell reinforcements, chemicals, and amino acids, making it an unimaginably reviving and wellbeing-advancing superfood. Spirulina is an ethical same.

Honey bee dust

With regards to youthful and delightful skin, honey bee dust has extraordinary gifts. Swedish dermatologist Dr. Lars-Erik Essen utilizes honey bee dust to effectively treat skin inflammation and other skin conditions and notices its enhancing and against maturing impacts.

He reports that honey bee dust 'appears to forestall untimely maturing of the phones and animates the development of new skin tissue. It offers successful assurance against parchedness and infuses new life into dry cells. It smoothes away kinks and invigorates a nurturing blood supply to all skin cells.'

He accepts its skin revival properties because of its high convergence of nucleic acids RNA and DNA, as well as its normal anti-infection activity. Honey bee dust has a large group of other wellbeing advancing advantages that incorporate battling contaminations, bringing down cholesterol, fortifying the blood, Boosting the insusceptible framework, expanding actual strength and endurance, supporting life span

furthermore, upgrading charisma! It has been known as a 'regent food' since it is so healthfully complete.

Coconut oil

Coconut oil speeds up your digestion and can assist you with free weighting. It is likewise staggeringly decorating and saturating for the skin and has cancer prevention agent properties that safeguard against free-extremist harm, keeping the skin energetic and solid

Taken inside or remotely coconut oil is an extraordinary partner for any excellent healthy skin system. It likewise contains lauric corrosive, an enemy of microbial unsaturated fat that kills microorganisms, infections, and organisms.

Section 5

Superfoods for a Super Long Life

Late exploration shows that particular synthetic compounds in food varieties - -, for example, sulforaphane, a phytochemical in broccoli - - work with your qualities to tighten up your body's regular safeguard frameworks, assisting with inactivating poisons and free revolutionaries before they can cause harm that prompts malignant growth, cardiovascular illness, and, surprisingly, untimely maturing.

Also, the expectation for what's to come is to have the option to let somebody know what illnesses or diseases they may be hereditarily inclined to right off the bat, so their weight control plans can be centered likewise.

We'll know which ones to add, which ones to keep away from and have the option to play a proactive job in forestalling or discouraging a hereditary illness. Meanwhile, numerous food sources are not entirely settled to sneak up all of a sudden into the maturing system.

Lycopene, the color that makes tomatoes red, additionally seems to lessen the risk for cardiovascular sickness, a few diseases, and macular degeneration. It's additionally been related to more noteworthy independence in older grown-ups.

Whilc ncw tomatoes have a decent hit of lycopene, the most absorbable structures are tracked down in cooked tomato items, for example, spaghetti sauce and soup and arranged salsas. Pink grapefruit, guava, red chime peppers, and watermelon are likewise wealthy in lycopene.

Eating no less than two cups of orange natural products like yams, squash and carrots support the admission of beta-carotene, which converts to vitamin A, fundamental for solid skin and eyes, and which may likewise decrease the gamble of certain malignant growths, cardiovascular infection, and osteoporosis.

Lutein and lycopene, likewise tracked down in orange produce, additionally assist with decreasing the gamble of macular degeneration and may shield skin from sun harm and even diminish wrinkling too. Mangos and melons are additionally beta-carotene invested.

Also, if you do nothing else to change your eating regimen, eat your dull mixed greens. They have been displayed to altogether decrease your gamble for coronary illness and may likewise save your visual perception. Dietary rules educate no less than three cups concerning greens seven days. Frozen or stowed is just about as great as new.

Remember the psychological maturing process by the same token. The heart-sound omega 3 unsaturated fats have additionally as of late been displayed to keep your mind sharp. A new report found that a higher admission of greasy fish fundamentally decreased cognitive deterioration. If new fish isn't a choice, go for canned fish, salmon, and sardines.

Section 6

Superfoods for Super Skin

It's been said we are what we eat, and that assessment surely turns out true to form concerning our skin.

It's our body's most prominent organ, and it justifies all the refreshing TLC we can give it. Along these lines, research what you've been dealing with yourself, and thusly dealing with your skin.

One of the fundamental pieces of skin prosperity is vitamin A, and probably one of its most remarkable wellsprings is low-fat dairy things. It might be said the sufficiency of our skin depends upon vitamin A.

Low-fat yogurt isn't only high in vitamin A, yet what's more acidophilus, the "live" microorganisms that are truly perfect for gastrointestinal prosperity. Winds up, it could in like manner influence the skin, since it assists with osmosis. Other incredible wellsprings of nutrient An integrate cod liver oil, sweet potatoes, carrots, verdant vegetables, and empowered breakfast grains.

It's basic to similarly guarantee you're eating food assortments well off in malignant growth avoidance specialists, similar to blackberries, blueberries, strawberries, and plums. The upsides of these food assortments for sound skin are bountiful. The cell fortifications and various phytochemicals in these normal items can defend the skin cells, so there is less of an open door for hurt.

This hence plans for inconvenient development and keeps skin looking young longer. Various results of the dirt that are high in malignant growth anticipation specialists consolidate artichokes, dull, red, and pinto beans, prunes, and pecans.

Basic unsaturated fats (EFAs) are urgent for your skin. Integrate salmon, walnuts, canola oil, and flax seed. EFAs keep cell films strong, and license enhancements to go through.

We furthermore need strong oils, which contain more than basic unsaturated fats. Eating extraordinary quality oils helps keep with tidying lubed up and keeps it looking and feeling much improved all around. Look for oils that are coldly crushed, similar to olive or extra virgin oil. We simply need around two tablespoons each day of strong oils, so use adroitly.

Selenium expects a critical part of the sufficiency of skin cells. Go to food assortments like Whole-wheat bread, rolls, and oats; turkey, fish, and brazil nuts for this huge enhancement. That is the thing continuous examinations show accepting selenium levels are high, even skin hurt by the sun may simply encounter immaterial, if any, hurt.

Picking the whole grain types of muddled starches can by and large influence insulin levels. Dealt with refined sugars can cause a disturbance that may finally be associated with skin breakouts.

Green tea has quieting properties, and it protects the film of the cell. It could help out thwart or decrease skin harmful development bets.

Water expects such a huge part of your overall prosperity, and it essentially influences your skin's prosperity as well. Overall hydrated skin is sound and energetic looking. It furthermore helps move the toxins out of your system so they have less an open door to hurt.

Section 7

Superfoods that Squash Stress

Life has an approach to outwitting us a few days. Whether it's functioning such a large number of hours, rearranging your children all over town for their exercises, dealing with your family, or managing individual or family matters, stress can negatively affect you genuinely, intellectually, inwardly, and profoundly.

However, there are basic advances you can take to battle pressure, beginning with the food varieties you eat.

Keeping away from caffeine and liquor is a decent beginning when life's especially unpleasant. Energizers and depressants like these can both zap your energy and deny you of the fuel you want to adapt to pressure effectively. Sweet food varieties ought to be stayed away from also, as they cause your glucose levels to spike then, at that point, plunge quickly, which can thusly make your energy levels spike and plunge at a similar rate.

Notwithstanding, there are a few superfoods out there that furnish you with the energy and nourishment your body needs to hold pressure in line

Asparagus, which is high in folic corrosive, can assist with evening out your temperaments. Folic corrosive and vitamin B are central members in creating serotonin, a substance that gets you into a positive state of mind.

Furthermore, however, we might hear negative things concerning red meat, it's a savvy supper choice for a worried family. Meat's elevated degrees of iron, zinc, and B nutrients not just assist with getting you into a positive state of mind, but, assist you with remaining there too. Your neighborhood butcher can assist you with choosing lean cuts for the best choices

Milk truly does a body decently. Packed with calcium, protein, cancer prevention agents, and nutrients B2 and B12, it fortifies bones and advances solid cell recovery.

Matched with a sound entire grain oat decision in the first part of the day, low-fat milk is an extraordinary method for beginning your day and arming yourself to fight with the

stressors that look for you. Curds are likewise one more extraordinary dairy decision, and when combined with an organic product that is high in L-ascorbic acid, it assists the body with combating free extremists that spin out of control during your most focused periods.

Almonds are likewise a marvelous decision with regards to equipping yourself against stress. They're high in magnesium, zinc, as well as nutrients B2, C, and E, and unsaturated fats, all of which are extraordinary heroes against free revolutionaries, which have been displayed to cause tumors and coronary illness.

www.ingramcontent.com/pod-product-compliance
Lightning Source LLC
LaVergne TN
LVHW052104160826
845678LV00015B/3357

* 9 7 9 8 8 4 6 9 9 0 9 9 9 *